Practical Way
of Managing Diabetes

Practical Way of Managing Diabetes

"Simple, Easy and Economical, Wherever You Live"

Chona M. Lobusta R.N., B.S.N.

To order additional copies of this book, contact:
Xlibris Corporation
1-888-795-4274
www.Xlibris.com
Orders@Xlibris.com
69371

Contents

Introduction 7

Chapter 1   Knowing Diabetes Management
             And Its Impact In Your Daily Life........................ 13
Chapter 2   The American Diabetes Association, Inc., 1996.............. 16
Chapter 3   The Difference Between Diabetes Mellitus
             And Diabetes Insipidus 19
Chapter 4   Understanding Your Diabetes And How To Monitor It......... 26
Chapter 5   Diabetes And The Risk Factors
             In The Development Of Diabetes........................... 31
Chapter 6   Hypoglycemia; Hypo; Low's Or Low Blood Sugar 37
Chapter 7   Ketoacidosis And Non-Ketotic Osmolar Coma................. 39
Chapter 8   Insulin And How To Administer Insulin Shots............... 41
Chapter 9   Glucagon Syringe... 49
Chapter 10   Adhering To Your Prescribed Treatment 52
Chapter 11   Foot Care 55

References and Reading 61

Introduction

Since I was a kid, I always love to read. I even wondered how Helen Keller wrote a book. I had read different kinds of books, but it frustrates me most of the time because I could not even remember the authors. I can always tell the whole story of that book, but unable to tell you who wrote it. Despite of my inability to remember the authors, still I am fascinated and admired them so much because of their capabilities, their guts and their motivations, above all their high intelligence that give them power to write. I even challenge myself if I can also write a short poem and out of my imagination I was able to write one and was able to recite it on stage during our school program.

When I entered high school, I started to have an interest in reading Prose and Poetry, however as I mentioned earlier, I would not remember who the authors are. I still wondered how those authors made their writings. So, in order to simplify my understanding, I decided to write my own book in order to make it easier for me to remember the author and no other than myself as the author.

One day, when I was in high school, our subject in a class is about "Writing". Our teacher gave us an assignment to write a poem. I became excited about the subject. I had an ambivalent emotion, in the sense that I like the subject, but I hate it because I don't know how I am going to start my own writing. Anyway, whether I like it or not, the writing must be done because this was to be submitted to our teacher the following day.

Next day, I submitted my written poem. Unfortunately my teacher was not happy about it because she thought I copied it from a book. In short, she marked it with a big capital letters: "THIS IS COPIED", "REPEAT". This means that I must write another one. My teacher was not satisfied and said to me verbally: "Because you copied this poem from a book, I need you to write your own". At my very young age of 15 years old, arguing with somebody especially my teacher is not my type, so without saying a word, I grab my writing pad and a pen, wrote a poem impromptu, which means, she asked me to write my assignment in front of her desk. At first, I was frustrated because I don't know how to start. It was difficult to think and start even a single word to write for the title of my poem. A few moments later, my brain started to work and my journey to reach the very end of my poem was accompanied by inspirations to finish my assignment and prove to my teacher that I can write my own poem.

Until at this very moment, I can still see myself how I wrote my poem from start to finish. With my head vowing down, looking at every pace of my right hand as I continuously move my pen into writing my poem, my teaching was sitting in her desk in front of me watching me constantly up to the finish line of my very own writing. I handed it to my teacher. I was a little bit nervous as I was standing in front of my teacher because before she glanced at it, then she looked at me straight to my eyes with her very own terrorizing eyes. If looks can kill, I guess I was already in the ground breathlessly. Can you imagine a teacher who looked at the student as if going to spank your behind? Well, that was my feeling at that time. I was thankful at that time that my teacher did not dare to spank me because if she did, my mom would be right there to rescue me. I felt that my teacher underestimated my very own intelligence quotient, but that was only for a moment and without saying a word, I turned my back headed for home.

When I entered pre-nursing school, taking up entrance exam was again traumatic because I thought that I would probably encountered the same thing as from my previous agonizing experience. However, I do realize that nursing is a different area of concern. In my opinion, writing ability is doing it using one's imagination to create the whole story of one thing to give satisfaction to the reader either real or unreal situation; unlike nursing ability is using one's critical thinking so you can move fast with precision in case of emergency situation such as saving one's life as in the a particular case of Diabetes. Whatever the differences of writing ability and nursing ability, I am still proud of myself because I passed the test. It boosts my confidence when my instructor congratulated me and I do believe in myself that I can do things that will give me the opportunity to succeed in my nursing career. I am on my way to the path of reaching my goal of educating people who suffers from a condition called Diabetes.

Continuing my nursing studies was a bit easy though. My English teacher in college was a very intelligent person. Although I was not good in speaking, probably because of my inferiority complex when I was young, besides, I guess, maybe I just talked that only me can understand what I am talking about. My teacher told me that I was excellent in writing and all I need to do is to practice my speaking ability. Do you think I was offended of what she said to me? Of course not. Definitely not at all. In fact, I took it as a piece of constructive criticism, a piece of advice that will improve my ability to face people, speak to them and ensure that I will be able to communicate to those people who need my help especially in giving health education. In fact, what my teacher said to me has always given me a window of opportunity to improve myself and boost my confidence.

One day, I dreamt of writing a book, but my dream never come to reality. Just because I don't know how to start, so it always ended up in fantasy. Anyway, I finished my bachelor of science in Nursing in 1981, passed the Board exam on the same year and got my professional license to work as a Registered Nurse. Due to some difficulty in finding a job in hospital-setting, I ended up working in a community health services. In other words, I was a community health nurse, which means I do traveling, conducting home visits and assess family's health needs. As a Community health nurse, it was my responsibility to give education to these people in the community. How I wish I could help them financially for them to pay for their Doctor's visits, buy their medications to treat their illnesses to further avoid the devastating effects or complications of diabetes. To make a big difference in their lives, I grabbed a piece of paper and a pen, wrote down the lists of my health teachings which they all appreciated.

It was a big challenge for me, when I encountered a diabetic man whose foot ulcer had been there for about a year. The foul smell of the wound almost suffocated me. The ulcer looks awful, nasty and black tissues were very visible to my naked eyes and a greenish stuff coming out from that foot wound.

I visited the place two times a week. When I came back for a home visit, I was carrying with me a big textbook in Medical Nursing by Brunner which until this very moment this book is still with me and some of its pages were already been eaten by the roaches, I guess. But mind you, this book is loaded with information on health teaching. I used the book as a reference guide to give health education in diabetes especially to this diabetic man with foot ulcer and to the family members as well. You see? It was worthwhile working in a community and it was very rewarding in my nursing profession. In fact, I never stopped giving health education because I strongly believed that it is beneficial to both young and adult who doesn't have an access to such education regarding health issues especially to those who has diabetes. On the other hand, community health nursing is a scary thing for me to do, because I was visiting places that were remote and very strange to me. Besides, I don't even know these people, but I think THE GOOD LORD put me in that position to help them, so I did it. It was also a hard work to do, but it was one of my fulfilling and satisfying experiences.

In my native land, Philippines few people have diabetes but most of these diabetic people remains undiagnosed and untreated due to unavailability of medical attention and because most of them ignore that they have this condition, others are due to lack of knowledge and to some others due to financial scarcity. Globally, diabetes is one of the most devastating conditions that affect the whole population and when remains untreated will make one's life miserable due to long term complications damaging all the important organs in one's body.

Nursing is a difficult task but it is still my passion and my great desire to formulate health teachings and write a book in order to expand my experience and in some ways, helping people worldwide especially to my home country, the Philippine islands, to manage diabetes and to create a positive outlook in life. Everybody knows that nursing is not an easy job but if you have the passion of helping people, this will at least lessen the difficulties in performing the job and responsibilities as a Professional health educator and as a nurse, in general. I am fully aware that nursing does not only mean dealing with people's health, but it is helping and healing one's life as a whole. A holistic approach is crucial in providing education in the management of any health condition such as Diabetes.

In this book, I am going to introduce to you one of the devastating diseases other known as Diabetes Mellitus, which is commonly called worldwide as Diabetes. Further, I am going to help and teach you on how you are going to manage it so you can live a happy life, enjoy every minute with your families and friends and above all living in this world with less worry and anxiety wherever you are. Furthermore, accompany it with a simple prayer to our Creator which is really my definite recommendation in everything you do, as it will also help you and guide you through as you continue reading this book. This book is a very valuable tool and is a powerful aid in preventing you from having the acute and chronic complication of Diabetes; however, we must always remember not to forget our Spiritual Guidance because there is no most powerful tool in healing except the Power of Prayer. If you put this book in your hands, you will be able to reach your goal to live a wholesome life despite of your Diabetes. I don't mean literally just to put it in your hands without reading it by heart, because this would become useless. You need to read this book and assimilate the contents so you will be able to reach your goal of having a healthy way of living. I also read few reference guides to help me give you more information on how to manage your diabetes in the best possible ways. This will definitely change your outlook in life. Don't give up. You have much more opportunity to be healthy and use this book as a simple tool guide. This is your starting point to live a good quality of life. Be healthy. Be happy.

Chapter I

KNOWING DIABETES MANAGEMENT
AND ITS IMPACT IN YOUR DAILY LIFE

Diabetes is one of the common problems worldwide. With the high technology, discoveries and researches made for diabetic medications and diabetic diets, it is sad to say that no one yet discovered a cure for diabetes. However, expert health care providers such as Diabetic Educator, Physicians and nurses can help in providing education in managing your diabetes. Your family physician is the right health care provider who will prescribe the best treatment for your diabetes and can even give you the health education and support and as a nurse, like me, it is my responsibility to enhance that support and continue the health education and teach you the nursing management in diabetes.

More and more people, young and adult have been discovered to have diabetes. Interestingly, but not surprisingly, emergency rooms and Doctor's offices have filled with diabetic people only to find out that either they have uncontrolled high blood sugar other known as hyperglycemia or abnormally low blood sugar other known as hypoglycemia. These are what we call the HI's and LOW'S in diabetes respectively. Hi's refer to high blood sugar and Low's refer to low blood sugar. Low blood sugar or hypoglycemia is the most common acute complication of diabetes especially if you are on insulin treatment and/ or on diabetic pills. There are also people who have wounds that never heals, infection sets in and sure enough, it is because of uncontrolled diabetes and no treatment had been given or the condition had been ignored for a long time.

Experience matters a lot and in my clinical experiences, I happen to know that people never died from diabetes but they actually died from devastating effects of its complications. As I mentioned earlier, one of the most common complication of diabetes is hypoglycemia or low blood sugar. This is an acute complication due to untoward effects of insulin therapy and/ or diabetic pills which lowers the blood sugar level. If you think about the logic of it, once the blood sugar is very low or no reading at all, this means that the body has no enough glucose or sugar content that circulate in the blood stream to feed the body system and to give nourishment to the brain in order to function normally which ended up in the loss of consciousness, finally coma and death if not treated immediately and properly. To prevent this condition to happen, I am going to teach you the simple easy way to manage your diabetes and for you to be able to live a normal life, eat the food you want and enjoy the everyday life and of course to make your everyday life easy, and a life that is better and happy.

If you are just aware of what is going on in your body and have the skills of managing your diabetes, it will help you to reduce your journey or trip to the hospital, ER, or clinics, above all it will be a cost effective way of managing your diabetes, which means reduced medical expenses. As you continue reading, notice that every word is written in a simple language and explanation in order for you to understand every detail of what I am trying to teach. Just remember that this book is not intended to treat, heal or cure your diabetes but this will definitely help you and guide you through in managing your diabetes wherever you go and whenever you are in desperate need of assistance especially when no licensed health care provider is available to help.

The existence of advanced technology, coupled with the skills and expertise of Doctors, enhanced by the great assistance, knowledge, skills as well as expertise of professional nurses and practitioners help all diabetic people to manage their diabetes. The additional support of the families, friends and loved ones, diabetic people will be able to function normally and confidently that they will be able to reach for help in case of emergency and in case that they may not be able to perform or act quickly to help themselves as a patient. Don't miss this opportunity to use my strategy in managing diabetes. This is your chance to make a big difference in your life. You can do it if you only look at the positive outlook in life.

Chapter II

THE AMERICAN DIABETES ASSOCIATION, INC., 1996

Let's talk about the result of my reading based on the 1996 American Diabetes Association Inc. If you noticed the year, it is 1996, however all the information found in this edition are very helpful guide in understanding your diabetes and how you can manage it. In my very sound and intellectual comprehension, this edition is an excellent reference guide and there is no difference whether you live in other part of the world, this is still a very helpful tool in managing diabetes. Explanation about diabetes, its signs and symptoms and the causes of hi's and low's are best expressed in a very simple and understandable language.

What about hyperglycemia? If your blood sugar is high this condition is called hyperglycemia. Hyperglycemia is one of the signs of diabetes, which over a period of time can damage your eyes, kidneys, heart, nerves and blood vessels. Signs and symptoms of high blood sugar include: headache, blurred vision, thirst, hunger, and upset stomach, and itchy skin, fruity smells on breathing, confusion and shaky, tired legs.

There are times that one may not be able to tell that the blood sugar is high. The best way to tell if blood sugar is high is to check the blood sugar level when those signs and symptoms occurred or being experienced by a person.

The blood glucose reading will tell you and help you decide on what to do. If you are not yet diagnosed as diabetic, my best recommendation is for you to have a quick visit to your Physician if ever you experienced those signs and symptoms as previously mentioned. It is only the physician who is licensed to diagnose your illness. Once the diagnosis has been made be sure to follow the advice of your Physician regarding the prescribed treatment. Obviously, if you have diabetes, you will be given a prescribed treatment such as diabetic pill or insulin or a combination of both therapies and it also depends upon the Physician and the seriousness of your diagnosis. Now, it is your turn to adhere to the treatment and continue monitoring your blood glucose level to prevent from adverse reaction of that medication which causes an acute complication which is very common when you are on diabetic pills, insulin therapy or a combination of both. Hypoglycemia is a common acute complication caused by any anti diabetic medications.

What is Hypoglycemia? Little or low blood sugar level is called hypoglycemia. This may occur after insulin use and/ or taking anti diabetic pills. If hypoglycemia is not treated properly and immediately, this can make you pass out and may even cause seizure, coma and even death. Most common causes of low blood sugar include: eating too little, skipping a meal or not eating at all, doing exercise that sweats you out and evidently taking too much insulin and taking anti diabetic pills. Sickness and alcohol also cause low blood sugar especially of course if you are already diabetic.

A person who has low blood sugar exhibits the following warning signs and symptoms: anxiousness, clammy, sweaty, clumsy, shaky, weak and tired, irritable mood, stubbornness, light headedness, headache, blurred vision, confusion, tremor and sleepiness. He may even become pale and hungry.

As further discussed in the 1996 American Diabetes Association Inc, there are two types of Diabetes. These are the type 1 diabetes and the type 11 diabetes. In Type 1 diabetes, there is no insulin or only a tiny amount of insulin is present in the blood, and the treatment of course is insulin therapy. Some people are born with type 1 diabetes, which means that an insulin treatment is needed for a lifetime. In Type 11 diabetes, the body has no enough insulin or has trouble in utilizing the use of insulin or both. The first line of treatment for type II diabetes is diet and exercise, in order to lose weight to a desired level. In cases that these two lines of defense failed, then an anti diabetic pills other known as hypoglycemic medications are needed to control diabetes. What will happen if these diabetic pills will not work alone? An insulin therapy will be added to your treatment. Bear in mind that when you are on diabetic medications, or insulin therapy and /or combination of both treatment you are vulnerable to have an acute complication of hypoglycemia due to the side effects of your treatment.

Determining the warning signs of hi's and low's of your blood sugar level will help you act quickly on what to do. I urge you to pay close attention to the guidelines as set by the American Diabetes association because this is one of the best helpful guides in managing your diabetes. Let everybody know that if uncontrolled diabetes is not treated, over a period of time, it will damage one's body organs, such as eyes, kidneys, heart and nerves that will lead to severe complications and finally death.

Chapter III

THE DIFFERENCE BETWEEN DIABETES MELLITUS AND DIABETES INSIPIDUS

Is it good or bad? A common question mostly asked by my patients when their blood sugar is being checked. These are the people who have Diabetes Mellitus. In lay man's term we call this condition Diabetes. Just remember that Diabetes Mellitus is very different from a Diabetes Insipidus. Interestingly, Diabetes Mellitus is popularly called by everybody simply and plainly as "Diabetes".

When I was in the Middle East, I encountered one patient who continuously drink water almost every hour and consumed a gallon of water every hour. Believed me, this was not a joke. She also urinates frequently but her intake of fluids is much larger than her output. At first, I was thinking she was just very anxious of something because she said she has big health issue about her diabetes. Out of my curiosity, I spoke to her Physician and told me that the patient has Diabetes Insipidus not Diabetes Mellitus. After that one case of diabetes insipidus, I had never encountered anybody who has that disease. Now we all know that Diabetes Mellitus is a. k. a. Diabetes.

In my understanding, let me define to you all, the difference between Diabetes Mellitus and Diabetes Insipidus. Diabetes mellitus is a disorder involving insulin while diabetes Insipidus involves ant diuretic hormones.

In order to make you understand a little bit more, I am going to share with you the difference between these two conditions which are backed up by my research of reading. According to G. Thibodeau; PhD and K. T. Patton, PhD: Diabetes Insipidus is a hypo secretion of anti diuretic hormone which is marked by extreme voiding of large volume of urine every day and the patient suffers from great thirst and dehydration in which the treatment requires the administration of anti diuretic hormone. Diabetes mellitus is a hypo secretion of insulin in which the treatment requires the administration of insulin. Clearly, you see the difference of these two entities.

As I mentioned earlier, Diabetes is a commonly used word for Diabetes Mellitus. When you hear a person says" I have diabetes" this means he or she has a problem with high blood sugar. If you are not sure of what he or she is talking about, just make it sure she is telling you about her blood sugar issues.

Diabetes affects both young and adult regardless of age, race and sex. Genetic factor or heredity plays an important role in having diabetes that is why children with diabetic parents are vulnerable to getting the disease. In a clinical setting you will see and observe that a diabetic patient has characteristic symptoms of excessive thirst, constant drinking and passing large amount of urine. These patients have uncontrolled diabetes.

There was a patient, he was a middle aged man, who reported upon history taking that before he was diagnosed to have diabetes, there was an incident that when he went for camping he peed on the soil under the tree and later on found out that a couple of ants are patrolling their way to the soil where he previously urinated. A bad habit of urinating on the ground but thanks to what he saw that prompted him to see his Physician and he was diagnosed to have diabetes. Weird thing happens and when it happens it is a call for help to treat the illness of diabetes, as in the case of this middle aged man.

According to the book: Living with diabetes by Dr. J., Gomez, the term diabetes is a Greek word for passing through because of the characteristic symptoms of unquenchable thirst, leading to constant drinking and passing large volume of urine. Dr. J., Gomez further stated that Diabetes Mellitus means honey-sweet and it was an Indian Doctor of the seventh century who first reported that the urine of diabetic person is sweet which is a very significant feature of this illness. Back to the story of a middle aged man who urinated on to the soil and a couple of ants were busy patrolling in the soil where he passed urine, this explains that those ants were attracted to the sweet smell and sweet taste of the urine.

Analyzing the theory and supported by the presence of the high blood sugar of this illness, the sweetness of the urine comes from the natural sugar or glucose that circulates in the bloodstream in excess, passing through the kidneys and ended up in urine. I think everybody knows that anything that is in excess is considered abnormal and this happens in diabetes that there is an excessive presence of sugar or glucose in the blood and urine.

Once the diagnosis is made that you have diabetes please do not ignore this illness. The treatment prescribed to you by your Physician is very important for you to adhere, to ensure that your diabetes will be under control. In fact a tight control is very crucial to prevent the occurrence of both acute and chronic complications of your diabetes. Taking your diabetic medications has pros and cons. It will control your diabetes; on the other hand it will give you the down side especially when it is not followed properly. Actually, all diabetic treatment will lower your blood sugar and that is the purpose of these prescribed treatments, to lower your blood sugar level. Your blood sugar will even drop to a zero number if you don't know how to follow the regimen. It will even cause you to pass out. All diabetic medications are called hypoglycemic medications. Hypoglycemic medication means medication that lowers your blood sugar. Once your blood sugar is low, it is called hypoglycemia and you have the so called Hypo's or Low's. Take note that our goal here is to maintain your blood sugar level to as nearly normal level as much as possible.

Hypoglycemia is most common to patients who are taking insulin. If hypoglycemia occurs a person will not be able to function, loss of consciousness ensues and death follows if remains untreated. Hypoglycemia is the most common side effect of taking anti diabetic/hypoglycemic medications, especially when on insulin injection. Be aware that hypoglycemia can be prevented. Early detection for any signs and symptoms of hypoglycemia will prevent from further complications such as brain injury and untimely death. It is crucial to learn on how to monitor your blood sugar using any available glucose meter, how to self administer insulin injection safely, comfortably and learn how to recognize the early warning signs and symptoms of hypoglycemia. Learning to do all these simple things will make a big difference in your everyday life. You can take action quickly in the matter of urgency and to help others who may experience the same situation as yours. Most of all let your loved ones know that you are diabetic and you can even share this book to them so they can help you too in times of your urgent health needs.

Recognizing the warning signs and symptoms of hypoglycemia is a top priority, because this will put your health in jeopardy when you don't know those signals. Many, many times when we are busy, we tend to forget to take a break and not taking snacks or even not eating meal or simply just skip a meal and plan to eat later. How many of us experience a feeling of being clammy and clumsy trying to finish our job to get to the deadline? Sometimes, we experience headache and lack of concentration to the work we are trying to finish or even to the point of being confused after a long period of fasting? Sounds familiar? Well, once you experienced these signs, it is time to take care of your body system, you need to feel and find out what your body needs, because your brain needs nourishment. If you are not diabetic, probably it is still okay. What about if you are diabetic? If you know how to manage your diabetes then you will know what to do.

Taking a meal or drinking something like milk, soda or orange drinks will surely make a big difference in your feeling. Feeling better and refresh and you are ready to go back to work again. It works like magic and all the headache, clumsiness and lack of concentration disappear. Taking analgesic for your headache might relieved you at some point but it is not strongly recommended, because if your headache is caused by low blood sugar that would not really help.

What about if you are diabetic? Is it okay to grab your pain killer to relieve your headache after a long period of not having food intake? No and Yes. No, in the sense that your headache might be caused by low blood sugar and yes, you can take pain killer maybe after checking your blood sugar making sure it is at least within the normal range. In this case, you are sure that the cause of your headache is not from the low blood sugar level.

Knowing the signs and symptoms of diabetes will prevent from the occurrence of devastating complication that will result in a permanent damage to different organs of the body or to a very untimely death. The key here is an early detection of those signs and symptoms of this illness and to help all diabetic people to receive the correct management of diabetes as well as to provide them with knowledge and skill in the self management to promote a good quality of life. Working as a nurse and dealing with diabetic patients has come to my knowledge and attention and these are proven facts that patient who has hypoglycemic episode presents these following signs and symptoms, such as sweating, cold clammy skin, being hungry, headache, sleepiness and very difficult to arouse from sleep. Others may appear confused, irritable for no apparent reasons and unsteady gait due to weakness. Some patients fall into a deep sleep and become unresponsive or unconscious. Presentations of all these symptoms need a prompt and immediate action to reverse the symptoms.

Dealing with your diabetes need a strong support system from family members, friends, and relatives or even from your neighbors. They need to know that you are diabetic. It is of high benefit to let them know on what to do in case you need them most. Help must always be available at the very moment you experience the episode of having a low blood sugar and these support system are the best and the right people who can help you. But how are they going to help if they don't know what to do? Well then, after reading this book spread your knowledge to these people or let them explore by themselves what is being written in this valuable book. I am sure this will be a very important tool not only in helping you in case of emergency but they will be able to help others who have diabetes like you.

There are different innovative approaches in self teaching and these can be applied in managing your diabetes. This does not mean that you need to prescribe your own treatment, but what you need is to choose the best approach which is cost effective, simple to follow and within your easy reach. Obviously enough, we are living in a computer age. Where everyone can use the internet in finding solution to a problem. Let us say, you want to know what diabetes is and how you are going to manage it, therefore surfing the internet is a way to do it. But what about if the internet is not available in your home? What if you could not afford to buy a computer or could not even afford to rent it? There are people who don't even know how to use the internet. If the internet in your area is free and always available that would be a good idea to learn without spending.

Let us move on to the next innovative approach, l like reading materials, such as text books and pamphlets. Reading materials is very helpful to acquire knowledge in managing your diabetes. Text book is much even better but are you going to buy a text book and read the whole text book? Besides this is also expensive? Participating in a research program could be also helpful in finding the solution to how effectively you can manage your diabetes, however, this strategy is of course time consuming and no one is interested to be a part of the research process, unless you are working in a laboratory research project.

What about visiting Doctor's clinics, nurse's offices and other qualified health care provider? I am not telling you not to visit your health care provider. What I am trying to emphasize, that if you are familiar on what to do about your illness, unnecessary journey to these places and to the hospitals can at least be prevented because every time you visit your physicians or other health care providers will cost you money and is also time consuming though it is worth it too, but every penny counts. Well, these are really the best way to do and a great help for you because Doctors, nurses are the qualified professionals who really can help you in guiding and teaching you the specific things you need for your diabetes. Are you happy to always go to these places every time you don't feel good with your diabetes? Come to think about it. If you give yourself a chance to learn the skills in managing your diabetes you will be able to avoid those unnecessary journeys. Do not let your diabetes empower you but let yourself have the power to control your diabetes. It is not too late to learn how you are going to take control of your diabetes. Be good to yourself by knowing how to deal with your diabetes but also be smart in spending your money for unnecessary hospital trips. Empower yourself to manage your diabetes.

Economy is scarce especially when facing a life threatening symptoms of any disease and if you are diabetic or on insulin therapy and/or on diabetic medication your risk of life threatening complication is very high, and if you don't know nothing of what is going on inside your body, your first thinking is to go to the hospital right away. However, if you can identify or recognize the early signs and symptoms of the acute complications of your diabetes you will be able to move quickly on what to do next thus avoiding unnecessary hospital journey. Remember, when you first diagnosed that you have diabetes, your physician had given you all the instructions on how to take your medications and the side effects of your medications and the nurse repeated the instructions for you. All you need to do is to adhere to what your physicians had ordered you to do and if it is not enough then this book is a sure guide for you to read and follow. I assure you this is a very easy, simple way to manage your diabetes wherever you live. Apply your knowledge, know the symptoms, apply your skills, give your management, and practice it every day and you are on your way to a better quality of life.

Chapter IV

UNDERSTANDING YOUR DIABETES AND HOW TO MONITOR IT

When I was in UK England, I decided to take up course in nursing management of diabetes. I was very proud and excited when my request to go to the university was granted by one of the prestigious hospitals in UK. It was a big plus because once the hospital sends a staff for study it is free of charge. Before I did this course, I already thought that this will be my best tool in dealing with diabetic people. Sure enough with the great support of the Diabetic nurse practitioner who of course is my intelligent and a very patient mentor, I did it and passed it with a satisfactory rating. Wherever I go I am very much confident that my knowledge, skills and expertise that I gained from UK will be used and I always use it in providing every diabetic patient the necessary information, health teachings and strategic approach in managing diabetes.

In the event that you feel completely confused on what to do, just take a deep breath, calm down and relax your mind. Don't panic and keep focus. You need your focusing power to the very life saving strategy to save your life or your loved ones in preventing the nasty complications of diabetes. All you have to do is just to continue on monitoring your blood sugar every day. In this way you will be able to track down your Hi's and Low's moments and you will be able to use the simple strategy that is found in this book.

Monitoring your blood sugar is the most important part in managing your diabetes. Just follow the simple, yet bullet eyed instructions. All you need is a small blood glucose machine. Any brand will do to measure your capillary blood sugar. A drop of blood is taken from the tip of your finger(s) and this is called the capillary blood. You can actually take a blood sample from other sites, like the ear lobe but it is much preferred to take the blood sample from the tip of the fingers. Aside from that is easier to do and it is less painful for you. Finger tips have lots of tiny vessels or capillaries that has good amount of blood supply.

There are many different kinds of Glucose meter available that you can buy. It is just all up to you which brand you want as long as it is convenient for you to use and affordable on your budget. You don't need an expensive glucose meter. What is important is the correct number that your meter is telling you. You can even carry this machine with you. Just put it in your purse or bag so you can always use it any time you need it. There is only one thing you need to do before using the glucose meter. It is crucial to do the quality control test of your meter, make it sure that it is correctly coded in accordance to the strips you are using so as to ensure that the correct result of the blood sugar is obtained. After doing this quality control test procedure your little machine is ready to use. There are also glucose meter available in the market that doesn't need to be coded, but cost wise this is a little bit expensive, however, I should say that this is worth to have it, because this is less work for you to do. To make it really accurate, always follow the accompanying literature with instructions provided by the manufacturer because this is very helpful in guiding you on how to use the meter correctly. Don't throw this literature away, because you will need this for the trouble shooting of your meter.

Now get ready with your meter. Before pricking your finger tip, start by washing your hands with mild soap and water. Mild soap is preferable because it will prevent your skin from too much dryness, otherwise your skin will breakdown especially if your skin is sensitive due to harsh ingredients of the soap. An alcohol swab can also be used to clean the area of your fingertip to remove any dirt, germs or bacteria at the surface of your skin. The key here is to keep the finger tip real clean eliminating any types of residue from the food you handle and reducing the presence of bacteria or germs. Touching food is normal but the sugar contents of the food or a glass of beverages that you touched will come in contact with your hands and finger tips. The sugar contents of your food stuff will give rise to a false reading of your blood sugar. As a constant reminder, always wash hands before pricking your finger tips or use an alcohol swab to cleanse your finger tip. Pat dry with a clean cloth or dry it gently with a clean cotton ball or clean tissue paper. Remember you are managing your diabetes at home or any where you are. You don't need to monitor your blood sugar in a sterile or aseptic technique but at least you must do it in a hygienic way. Hand washing here is for cleansing, removing any glucose contents of any food stuff that contaminate your hands and fingers and of course for infection control reason.

The sides of your finger tips are the most commonly used areas in obtaining a drop of blood sample due to the fact that it is rich in capillary blood supply. According to most diabetic people these area are also less painful. Using your meter lancet, prick quickly but gently the side of your finger tip. I remembered most of my patients would tell me: "Please do it in the very side of my finger tip because it is less painful". If you are diabetic, I am sure you feel the physical pain and even the emotional impact especially if you are not ready or prepared to accept the reality that you have diabetes.

For me, it is very challenging in dealing with the physical pain, that I inflicted to my patients through pricking their finger tips, that it taught me how to be compassionate, showing my empathetic as well as sympathetic attitude to these precious individuals who entrusted their lives to my professional, yet gentle loving care that they deserved. Being compassionate, empathetic and sympathetic with the gentle approach of caring will also lessens the anxieties and worries in dealing with these people and in turns reducing their pain level.

Pricking the finger tips of my patients is my daily routine. I also happen to observe that these diabetic people continue to perform their activities of daily living, such as going to the bathroom, flushing toilet seats, picking things or handling things they need, like pens and paper as they write notes to families and friends and other kinds of activities of daily living. With my piece of common sense, I decided to make a difference in performing the prick. I thought that it is not wise to prick the forefinger and the thumbs. I strongly recommend using the middle finger, ring finger or the pinky. It is preferable, healthy wise, not to prick the thumbs and forefingers, in the sense that these are the most parts that are always used to touch things, pick up things and designed to perform almost all the activities of daily needs. Avoidance of pricking these two areas will prevent the further entry of unexpected infection that will come in contact with the skin opening that was previously pricked.

By squeezing the finger tip gently, apply a drop of blood on to the glucose strip which was already inserted in the glucose meter. In few seconds the reading of your blood sugar will appear at the window screen of the glucose meter machine. Having your knowledge about diabetes will determine your ability to tell what is a normal blood sugar level and what is not and will help you decide on what to do next or what action you need to take.

How bad or how good is your blood sugar level? Do you know what is within normal limits or the acceptable limits of your blood sugar? Blood sugar can also be checked from a blood sample obtained from any other route, for example the one that was taken from intra venous or veins. Here, you are not going to take blood from your veins Okay? But let us talk specifically the capillary blood that is taken from the very tips of your finger. This blood drop is obtained from the small vessels known as capillaries which supplies good amount of blood found at the vey tip of fingers that is why we call it capillary blood and when the result of the blood sugar comes up then we call it capillary blood sugar or CBS. If you know that your capillary blood sugar is normal, then you don't have to worry about it. What about if you don't know? Most of the time, people with diabetes will ask: Is it normal?" "Do I need to take my pills?" "You think I need my insulin?". Actually, most of the people with long term diabetes know exactly when to take their insulin shots or pills. However, there are times that these people are just feeling frustrated about their condition and that is why, it is the role of the health care provider to provide them the health teachings they need. Other diabetic people just want a confirmation that they are doing the right thing for their diabetes.

Basically, a blood sugar level needs to be checked before each meal that is before breakfast, before dinner time, before supper time and at bed time and even at 3 am. The normal range of blood sugar level before any meal is 80-120 mg/dl; at bedtime it is 100-140 mg/dl and at 3:00 AM 80 mg/dl or over, (American Diabetic Association Inc.). Take control of your diabetes and when you know the normal values of blood sugar it will be much easier for you to take action when needed.

It is crucial to adhere to the instructions that your Physicians told you to follow when you're taking diabetic treatment. Do not try to change the dosage of your medications without consulting your attending Physician. It would be a biggest mistake in your life if you try to change the dosage of your medicine because you will end up of not getting enough or you will be getting more which is very dangerous to your health. If you are not sure of what to do with your medication, I urge you to consult your Physician.

Unfortunately, there are diabetic people who are solely dependent from taking medication hoping that their diabetes will be treated permanently. They never came to realize that it can only be controlled. Others are ignoring their diabetes because they are confident that their medications will completely cure their diabetes. Bear in mind that there is no permanent cure for diabetes. Have you ever heard of pancreas transplant? Well, I am not sure about this transplant because I had not witnessed anyone who undergone such procedure to treat diabetes permanently. I honestly say that keeping your blood sugar under control is the only way that all of the devastating effects of complications can be avoided.

Chapter V

DIABETES AND THE RISK FACTORS IN THE DEVELOPMENT OF DIABETES.

According to the Merck Manual of Information, Diabetes Mellitus is a disorder in which the blood glucose level is abnormally high because the body does not produce enough insulin. There are two types of Diabetes Mellitus and these are Type 1(formerly called Insulin—dependent diabetes or the Juvenile onset diabetes) and Type 2(formerly called Non-insulin—insulin diabetes or Adult onset diabetes).

Whatever the type of diabetes a person has, it is crucial to be aware that this disorder needs to be managed and controlled. People with diabetes needs to know the risk factors to prepare themselves on how are they going to deal with this disease in case they will have it and to avoid those risks that can be avoided.

Diabetes is a hereditary condition. It handed down from parents to children. Children with both parents who are diabetics are at increased risk of vulnerability. A person would be lucky enough not to have diabetes when parents have it. There is nothing we can do about this inheritance, but it is very important to know our hereditary components so we can always prepare on how to deal with it or do something about it. Besides, it would help us avoid other risk factors that can contribute to the development of diabetes.

Heredity or not, once you got diabetes you need to accept it in order to manage this condition effectively and live your life to the fullest. Being aware of the genetic factors will help a person guards against the risk.

Healthy diet will lower the risk of diabetes. Food low in fats will lower the risk for both diabetes and heart attack. Carbohydrates and fibers are good for diabetes too. Avoid foods that are high in sugar contents such as refined sugar and chocolates. These kinds of food will surely stimulate sugar or glucose productions in your system or blood stream giving rise to a high blood sugar level. Take all things in moderation.

Eating too much will make you fat or grossly obese or over weight. As we grow older, it is very hard to loss the unnecessary weights. Modification of diet or choosing the right food to eat will help a person lose weight. Continuing eating unhealthy foods especially high in sugars and fats will not only contribute to overweight but you will also be at risk of developing diabetes, hypertension, stroke and heart attack. Have you noticed an overweight person? They tend to be lazy and unable to perform activities of daily living because they have difficulty in moving around due to the heaviness of their overweight body. If you are overweight you tend to be lazy most of the time, prefer to sit down, watching TV program or just sleep and doing nothing except eating. You even become depressed because you don't know what to do about your weight and the only thing you want to do is to adhere to your comfort zone of eating. You become even addicted to food, making you eat more and more instead of doing positive things or doing something for your weight.

Don't know what to do about your weight? Here is the first thing you need to do before it is too late. Instead of just sitting down in your comfortable chair, or eating your comfort food all the time, you need to jump start of getting up. Move, stand up, stretch your body and start walking. EXERCISE, EXERCISE, EXERCISE. Walking for at least 30 minutes every day is a form of active exercise. Be active and be healthy. Walking will give a huge difference in your weight an in your outlook in life. It will help you lose weight. If you don't move what will happen? You become more and more over weight, depression strikes and it attacks you every minute of your day. In fact when you are overweight, you tend to lower yourself esteem too. Furthermore, you will lose the courage to face and deal even the normal family problems that occur in your daily life. Once you are faced with any kind of situations, the stress is very high that you become vulnerable to have depression all the time. Do not wait until stresses and worries strike and it becomes difficult and too late for you to manage. So make your body moves, sweat it out, do not hibernate, perform your exercise and start living a happy life thus avoiding the risk of diabetes.

A diabetic person has a very low immune system which makes them vulnerable to the development of many kinds of infection, especially viral infection. Wound healing is also very slow and infection can easily sit in.

As I continue working and dealing with diabetic and non diabetic patients, I have learn and observed that there are medications that triggers the rise in blood sugar level. Steroids, Phenytoin and even diuretic medications can trigger high blood sugar levels even to some patients who are not diabetic. Most of these non diabetic patients will ask: "Why my blood sugar is is high and I am not diabetic?" At least a simple explanation is needed to let them understand that those medications as mentioned trigger the rise in their blood sugar temporarily while they are still on those medications. What about if you are diabetic and at the same time you are taking steroids, or diuretics or phynetoin? The chance of getting a high blood sugar level is very high, but taking precautionary measures is a must and you need to monitor your blood sugar very closely to ensure a tight control of your diabetes. Some of my patients reported that they acquired diabetes because they had taken steroids although they have no family history of diabetes. Remember your genetics? Think of the possibility that your parents might not have diabetes but your close relatives, an aunts or an uncle's has this illness so this is still considered as a part of your genetic components.

No one cares about ourselves when we were still young. At a very young age we seemed to be healthy and never worry at all of what is coming up in our future health, because we always feel good, but as we grow older our immune system becomes vulnerable to different kinds of health issues then we came to realize that having a family history of diabetes makes one vulnerable to have diabetes. One day, after visiting your physician for next routine check up, it happens that your blood sugar was high and finally you were diagnosed with diabetes. So you see, as we grow older we need to watch every single thing that is happening in our body, because age is one of the risk factors in developing diabetes. Sad to say, no one can avoid the aging process.

Although genetics play an important part in the development of diabetes, interesting but not surprisingly, no professional health care provider will advise any woman not to become pregnant. I had seen a lot of diabetic women who were pregnant and were able to deliver a healthy baby. A close follow up with their pregnancy is needed to tightly control their diabetes. They even delivered their babies with no complications at all. Some women delivered a large baby, but a C section is advised to avoid complications to both the mother and the baby. I witnessed several women who delivered their babies via C section because their babies are bigger than average babies that are impossible to come out to the new world via normal delivery. If you are planning to get pregnant or if you are on your pregnancy, first and foremost is to keep monitoring your blood sugar tightly and always keep it within normal or as close to normal range as much as you can.

Controlling your diet will play a major role in the prevention of rapid gain weight during pregnancy period. Eating healthy diet is essential to contribute to the well being both for you and your baby. Always remember that the source of nourishment of your baby depends on what you are taking in.

Smoking is other risk factors when you have diabetes especially when you are pregnant. Better quit smoking to promote the good health of both of you and your baby.

Check your blood sugar frequently. How frequent? Checking blood sugar needs to be done at least every before each meal, 2 hours after meals and at bedtime. Even if your blood sugar is stable, I do recommend checking your blood sugar in the early morning especially when you are on insulin injection. Patients may experience either the Somogyi phenomenon in which the patient becomes hypoglycemic during the night or the morning hyperglycemia in which the blood sugar becomes high upon awakening., (All-In-One., Resource Care Planning by Mosby, 2004). I observed that most of the patients experience a drop in their blood sugar that happens sometimes in the middle of the night and 3 o'clock in the morning and most of these patients are on insulin injection. This syndrome is called Somogyi phenomenon. This can also be avoided by taking a bedtime snacks such as a cup of milk, an orange juice or some crackers. There are also cases that blood sugar becomes high in the morning upon awakening or earlier before breakfast then we call this as Dawn phenomenon. So if you are on insulin therapy, make it sure to check your blood sugar early in the morning when you wake up because you might need your insulin shot. If you experienced either of these phenomena, you need to tell your Physician for possible adjustment of your diabetic medications or insulin injections.

If you are pregnant you need to see your OB-Gynecologist physician. Check out on scheduled visits to monitor your pregnancy. Make it sure that your urine is also checked for the presence of glucose and acetone. You can even check your urine at home using a glucose strip for urine which you can buy it over the counter without any prescription at all. You might be advised by your physician to take insulin injection. Your physician is responsible to give the right treatment of your diabetes. Never take insulin shots without checking first your blood sugar. Why? Taking insulin by not knowing your blood sugar is dangerous because you may end up with hypoglycemia which is a devastating complication due to adverse effects of your diabetic treatment.

If a woman becomes pregnant, the physician might put her on insulin therapy instead of taking diabetic pills. It is only the physician who can change the treatment of diabetes. A 3o minutes walking exercise is advised for a pregnant person instead of vigorous exercise. Walking will not only help a person lose weight, in fact it can increase endurance and build up strength. It can also burn the excess fats and sweats out those toxins present in the body system. A well balanced diet is very important for both the mother and the growing fetus. Of course an increase in water intake is needed. Normally, 6 to 8 glasses of water is needed by us every day but more than this is needed during pregnancy period. Drinking water can help flush the toxins out of the body and it will even get rid of the ketones out of the body system.

Everybody especially pregnant women, need to be aware that the presence of ketones in the urine and blood is highly dangerous especially during pregnancy. Testing urine for the presence of ketones will definitely help the pregnant women to avoid the life threatening situation of diabetes.

Ketone testing can be done any time every day. This is a very easy and simple procedure using a test strip. A urine sample can be applied directly to the strip or can be dipped to urine then read the result in just few seconds or a minute depending on the instructions on how to read your strips. Compare the result from the color chart found in a test kit and it will give you the final result. For accurate result always follow the guidelines accompanying the test strip kit. If you have difficulty of doing this procedure, a nurse or a physician can help you on how to test your urine for ketones properly. The presence of ketones in urine indicates an urgent and prompt attention because ketoacidosis will occur in just a couple of hours that it needs an urgent treatment or hospitalization. Contact your Physician immediately for further management of your diabetes, Ketone testing kit can be bought over the counter in any drug store or pharmacy. You don't need a prescription for this test strips.

The Physician can also give the meal plan needed for pregnancy. A dietician also is the best health care provider who can assist on healthy eating plan.

Chapter VI

HYPOGLYCEMIA; HYPO;
LOW's OR LOW BLOOD SUGAR

Hypoglycemia is called low blood sugar. Other people call it as Hypo's or Low's. Hypoglycemia is a frightening situation in diabetes. This condition needs urgent treatment before a person becomes unconscious. When low blood sugar is not treated urgently and promptly it will lead to most serious complications such as coma and finally death. I had never encountered a person who died from diabetes itself but a person dies from a serious complications of diabetes. Acute or chronic complications of diabetes have debilitating effects to the overall health of an individual.

A person may experience warning signs and symptoms of hypoglycemia. In a clinical setting, I gathered almost all patients who experiences hypoglycemia have the same responses and exhibited these following symptoms: cold clammy and sweating, clumsiness, light headedness, headache, and nervousness, sick to the stomach, sometimes angry and anxious without apparent reason, irritability and drowsiness. Finally, the person feels sleepy eventually becomes unresponsive. If these symptoms remain untreated death may follow.

If you have diabetes it is very important to keep anything sweets either in your pocket, purse or in your car, and always have a ready to drink or eat snacks to alleviate hypoglycemia. A glucose gel and a glucose tablet are available over the counter in the pharmacy and you need to store these items in your house or in your car and these can be easily taken by mouth. For a Glucose gel, you can just open the tube and squeeze the desired amount of gel direct to your mouth. If you are giving this gel to other diabetic person, make it sure that the person is fully awake to prevent from choking. You can also rub the gel onto the gums and it will be absorbed quickly. Most of the glucose gels are low in sodium or no sodium contents at all and this is good for people who are on low sodium or no sodium diet. Gels are also good for hypertensive people who are avoiding salt intake and it comes in different flavors too. Glucose tablets can be dissolved in water and drink it straight. Glucose tablets also come in different flavors to suit your taste. At bedtime, it is very important to take a bedtime snacks especially when taking insulin to prevent hypoglycemia that usually happens at midnight or in the early morning. An orange drinks or milk can be taken before going to bed.

What causes hypoglycemia? Taking insulin shots. Oral hypoglymic pills, alcohol, excessive exercise, skipping a meal or not eating at all contribute to a hypoglycemia. A person needs to be treated urgently. What to do in case of low blood sugar depends entirely on how knowledgeable you are in dealing with this emergency situation. There are times that low blood sugar occurs without the signs and symptoms being noticed even by yourself that you are unable to get the immediate treatment for yourself. I written this book to be available not only for you as a diabetic person but also for your loved ones, family and friends for them to read and learn and apply their knowledge and skill and put this into practice to help you in case of diabetic crisis occurs.

This could be a guiding tool for everybody to apply the strategies in managing diabetes in a calm and effective way.

Chapter VII

KETOACIDOSIS AND NON-KETOTIC OSMOLAR COMA

Ketoacidosis is a very dangerous complication in which the body metabolism is in jeopardy due to lack of insulin. In Type 1 diabetes ketoacidosis can quickly develop and without insulin, fat cells begin to breakdown producing compound called ketones and making blood more acidic. As the ketone escapes through breath. The smell of the person's breath is like a nail polish remover called acetone. In Type 11 diabetes, ketoacidosis does not usually develop due to the presence of some insulin. But blood sugar level can become extremely high due to some stressors like infection and drug use. Severe dehydration develops which may lead to mental confusion, drowsiness and seizures, a condition known as non ketotic hyperglycemic hyperosmolar coma. (THE MERC MANUAL of MEDICAL INFORMATION). When a patient has ketoacidosis. acetone and ketones are present in the blood as well as urine. However there are cases that ketones are not usually present and the person can still develop a diabetic non ketotic hyper osmolar coma. Some types of medicine, for example, steroids can trigger the extremely rise in blood sugar level. If you are taking medications like this type, you need to monitor your blood sugar closely to ensure that it is tightly controlled.

Signs and symptoms of ketoacidosis include dry mouth, excessive or great thirst, and stomach pain nausea and vomiting, dry flushed skin, frequent urination, fruity breath smell, labored breathing and drowsiness ;(American Diabetic Association Inc). Knowing all these signs and symptoms will help you understand what is happening inside your body. In fact, if you are diabetic and knowledgeable about your diabetes, once you feel or experience these signs and symptoms, you will be able to act quickly and promptly on what action you need to take.

You can actually tell when a person is in ketoacidosis. When I was a student I had a patient that when I entered in her room, I smelled something like an acetone. While I was talking to her, I noticed that I can smell her acetone breathe. Although she was breathing normally, I noticed that her lips appeared dry and she was constantly drinking few glasses of water. I also observed that she kept on going to the bathroom and she complained of excessive and frequent urination. Frequent and excessive urination can make a person dehydrated. She was fully awake, well oriented to everything but she said that she felt weak and sleepy. Knowing that she was a diabetic patient, I immediately checked her blood sugar and it only says "Hi" in a glucose meter. This patient was immediately seen by the Physician and was given an urgent treatment. These are the typical signs and symptoms of a diabetic ketoacidosis that if not treated promptly and quickly can threaten the life of a person. It doesn't matter what type of diabetes you have, what matters is that, once your blood sugar is extremely high, this is an emergency situation that an urgent treatment is necessary to save your life. When the treatment is not administered immediately, it will even cause death.

Try to look back at the signs and symptoms exhibited by my patient. An acetone smell on her breath, dry lips/mouth, frequent and excessive urination, excessive thirst, feeling weak and sleepy. These are the typical signs and symptoms of extremely high blood sugar with ketoacidosis and the patient doesn't even know about it. What do you think will happen if she is not in the hospital? I bet you know it. So if you are diabetic, knowledgeable, able to recognize those signs and symptoms, it would be easy to manage your diabetes even you are at home or where ever you go.

Chapter VIII

INSULIN AND HOW TO ADMINISTER INSULIN SHOTS

Aside from monitoring your blood sugar level and taking oral hypoglycemic tablets or diabetic pills, a self insulin injection is an important part of managing your diabetes. Insulin syringes are usually calibrated in "IU" or International unit. You need to know how to read the calibration to ensure that the correct dose of insulin is administered to your body. Delivering too high or too low of insulin is very dangerous. Too much insulin will put you at risk of having very low blood sugar known as hypoglycemia. On the other hand, if you receive less insulin your blood sugar will remain too high other known as hyperglycemia and your diabetes will not be controlled, which in over a period of time it will have a bad or dangerous impact to your overall health damaging the most important organs of your body, such as eyes, heart, nerves, kidneys and even your skin.

Have you ever wondered if there are people who are allergic to a certain kind of insulin? There are people who are said to be allergic to pork and beef, which means that they can only receive human insulin preparation. Interestingly, in my entire career, I only knew one person who has allergy to a certain type of insulin made from beef and pork. Unfortunately, I could not tell you exactly how this person reacted because I did not witnessed it by myself. I just happened to know it by taking his medical history and the

Physician prescribed that "only human insulin be given". I also heard some Doctors saying that there are also patients who are allergic to human insulin but so far I have not seen or encountered anybody having adverse reaction to human insulin. This is a very rare case; however, it is very crucial for everybody to be honest in telling your professional health care provider about your medical history to give your Physician the opportunity to provide you with the best care you deserved and the correct treatment for your diabetes. Remember that the success of your treatment depends on the detailed information you provide to your Physician. It is you who knows your body more than anybody else in the world. So be honest in telling your medical history to your Physician.

Learning to self inject insulin is very easy. It only needs a very little effort and confidence in performing this simple task. You can also try something different in learning how to do it. For instance, a piece of apple or a piece of orange fruit instead of using a dummy which is expensive. Practice holding your insulin syringe and inject it to the soft skin of an apple or an orange fruit. You can also try to use the whole tomato but choose the one that is not too ripe. Sounds silly, but it is okay to try different things if it has the benefit to your learning process. Believe me, it works. Practice your hand coordination while your handling the whole tomato and injecting your insulin syringe direct to the skin of tomato. Isn't it your skin is soft? So with the skin of tomato. Don't pinch or hold the tomato tightly or else its skin will break open and the flesh will splash on to your face. The same thing as when you hold your skin, you need to be gentle too. This could be your innovative approach in learning how to self administer insulin.

The first time I did my nursing job, I was nervous and hesitant to give insulin injection to my patient, because I was not confident enough to do it. Until one day, I decided to practice in an orange fruit. The skin of an orange fruit is a bit harder and bumpy, so I decided to use an apple fruit. An apple fruit is okay, although the skin is smooth, its flesh is a little bit hard as well. My last recourse was to use the tomato and I finally did it successfully. Folks, this sounds funny, even scholars or any clever teachers will not tell you to do it, but this really works for me. It might work for you too. This method is a fun way of learning and will help you do the trick to confidently self inject your insulin. Why pay The high cost of medical expenses and pay someone just to administer your insulin if you can practice and do it to yourself with ease and confidence. Learn and apply it into practice and practice will always make you perfect. All you need is your willingness to learn and help yourself. As long as you pay attention to detail of what you need to know and learn, you health will always be in top shape. In this way, it will even prevent you from unnecessary trip to hospitals or clinics just to have a nurse or doctor administer your insulin. Be a good teacher to yourself. Wherever you live or wherever you go, just carry your insulin kit and whenever you need help, you can always help yourself to inject your own insulin. So you see? Your knowledge, skills and expertise, coupled with courage and a little effort in self insulin injection and your preparedness of what action to take will always save your life.

There are diabetic people who use insulin pump. This is a small machine and a syringe with a gear driven plunger and a needle. The syringe is filled with required insulin, positioned inside a machine and a needle is inserted into the skin. Needle can also be inserted to the thigh or abdomen. Most patients preferred to insert it in the abdomen for ease and comfort. It is much comfortable for them to carry and keep it steady under their clothes, but just the same, inserting a needle into your skin needs skill too. The only difference is that the needle of the insulin pump does not need to be inserted to the skin every day for several times except when the syringe is empty where as insulin syringe injection are done several times every day. The insulin pump needs to be programmed on how much insulin a person should be getting and this will really control tightly the blood sugar level. Always remember that whatever method you are getting for an insulin treatment, a close monitoring of your blood sugar needs to be done always. Never, rely on insulin alone without monitoring your blood sugar.

Do you know where to administer your insulin shots? You are not going to inject the insulin in any areas that you want. There are designated sites in your body where you must need to inject your insulin shot. These areas are in the abdomen, thighs, lateral parts of the upper arms and buttocks. Buttocks are rarely used. Well, I am sure you will not inject your insulin in your buttocks because if you are fat you will be having difficulty of reaching and looking at the right spot, anyway. If you can reach your buttocks then that is fine, just do it if you feel comfortable doing it. Beneath the skin of these areas are rich in adipose fatty tissues.

Breakfast and lunch insulin can be injected in the arms and abdomen because the insulin absorbs faster in these areas, while the supper and bedtime insulin doses can be injected in the buttocks and thighs which give slower insulin absorption and it is recommended to inject insulin one inch apart from each injection site to prevent tissue damage. (The American diabetes association Inc.) If you are doing self injection, your only preferred areas are absolutely your upper arms, thighs and abdomen because it would be impossible for you to reach your buttocks, right? But if you are administering the insulin shot to another diabetic person, you can choose the upper arms, buttocks, thighs and abdomen.

When I worked in an endocrinology clinic I had seen patients who are diabetic and their skin in the thighs and abdomen appear, wrinkled, lumpy, bumpy, wavy and hard to touch. These are the areas where they inject their insulin and administering it in the same areas every time insulin was given. This is called a lipodystrophy where there is fatty tissue damage. There is a loss of body fats and redistributed it to other areas of the skin which causes a bumpy area on your skin. Always rotate the injection site to prevent the development of lipodystrophy. In lipodystrophy there is the local disturbance in fat metabolism resulting in the loss of fat or the abnormal presence of fatty masses at the injection sites, (All-In-One., Care Planning Resource by Mosby, 2004).

But this condition rarely happens due to the knowledge and the health education provided by the health care professional to the diabetic persons and the hundred percent compliance of the diabetic people to follow instructions will prevent the occurrence of tissue damage.

ILLUSTRATIONS BELOW SHOW THE AREA WHERE TO GIVE THE
INSULIN SHOTS:

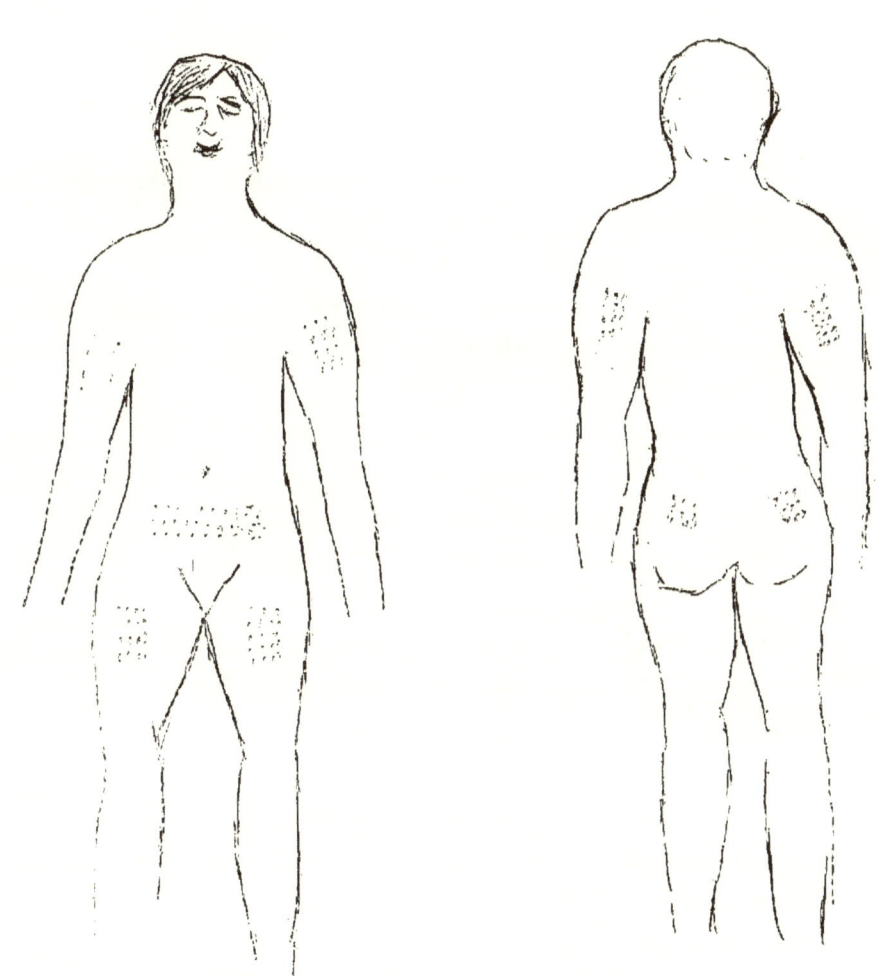

Sites for Insulin injection
Dots represent the site for injection

RED DOTS REPRESENT THE AREAS WHERE TO INJECT THE INSULIN SHOTS

Always choose a new sites when giving the next dose of insulin to prevent tissue damage, (Nursing Procedure made incredibly easy, Springhouse; 2002).

Steps in administering Insulin Injection:

1. Wash hands with mild soap and water. Dry hands with clean cloth or towel. Hand washing will prevent the spread or cross infections.

2. Using alcohol swab or 70 % isopropyl alcohol, wipe the top of the insulin vial.

3. Insulin vial comes in either clear or mixed solution. Mixed solution appears somewhat whitish, milky color.

    When it comes in a mixture solution, gently roll the vial in between your hands until the mixture is well blended or well mixed. Avoid shaking the bottle vigorously. If the solution comes in crystal clear there is no need to roll the vial.

4. With one hand, turn the vial upside down. Insert the needle with syringe into the rubber top of the vial and draw insulin, then stop at the mark for the amount of unit you need.

    You can inject air into the vial equivalent to the amount of insulin you need before you finally draw the insulin solution into the syringe. Injecting air into the vial of insulin will create a vacuum in drawing the insulin, besides it is much easier and quicker to draw the insulin.

5. After drawing insulin into the syringe, check for the presence of air bubbles. Get rid of the air bubbles by holding the syringe in upright position with needle pointing in upward position, and tapping the syringe gently or flicking it with your finger.

6. Choose the area where you want to inject the insulin. Clean or wipe gently that chosen area with alcohol swab or 70% isopropyl alcohol.

   This alcohol swab or isopropyl alcohol can be bought over the counter or without prescription at all. Cleansing the area where you want to inject the insulin will remove the bacteria or germs that might be present at the surface of the skin preventing it from entering the punctured or the injection site, thus controls infection.

7. Now gently grasp a fold of that skin. Holding the syringe with your other hand, just like as you are holding a pen to write, then inject the needle into the skin in right angle position.

   When doing this procedure, you need to keep your hand steady and inject the needle quickly into the skin and push the plunger of the syringe gently to introduce the insulin solution into the fatty tissues. It is much less painful when you insert the needle quickly and introduce the solution gently, than to insert the needle slowly into your skin.

9. Remove the needle and apply a gentle pressure to the injection site using an alcohol swab for at least 5-8 seconds.

   You don not need a watch to time it per second. All you need is to count it mentally from one to five or eight. Say these: One and two and three and four and five. Each count represent one second. So you see how easy it is. A gentle pressure in that injection site will prevent the possible slight bleeding to that punctured site and also it will help the insulin solution be distributed evenly into the fatty tissues.

10. Discard the used insulin syringe and needle into an appropriate container. Its disposal must always be done properly. It is dangerous to place any used insulin syringes and needles to a garbage cans or bins without securing them in a well sealed and punctured—proof container because of the possibility of accidental prick injury to others or even to yourself.

If someone is punctured with a used needles, that person will always be at a higher risk of acquiring a blood borne infectious disease, such as hepatitis and AIDS. To prevent this from harming others, always dispose your used needles and syringes in a safe, sealed punctured resistance container. An improvised sharp container will do the trick, for example, an empty soda cans or a thick plastic container or bottles, sealed it securely before finally throwing it into the garbage bin. In this way, everyone is going to be safe and be able to prevent from sharp or needle injuries.

STORAGE OF INSULIN SOLUTION VIALS:

Always follow the instructions of the insulin makers or companies on how to store your insulin vials. Almost all of the insulin companies or insulin makers will recommend that the insulin solution vials be stored in a refrigerator and these are not to be stored in a freezer or in any environment of extreme heat. However, it can be stored at room temperature for only a short period of time without affecting its potency. Once the insulin vial is opened, you need to write the date and this should be stored in a refrigerator. This can be also being stored at room temperature and be used for a month without destroying the insulin potency as recommended by ADA.

Chapter IX

GLUCAGON SYRINGE

Glucagon releases glucose into the blood stream causing blood glucose to rise thus alleviates hypoglycemia. Glucagon comes in a syringe with accompanying leaflet instructions. If you have glucagon at home or with you, try your best to read and understand the instructions on how to use it and also, let your family, friends or loved ones know how to use it for you. Your physician can give this prescription for you and you can keep it at home or carry it with you if you like. As I've said. Let others know how this glucagon be used for you in case you are unable to do it for you.

If you have a critical low blood sugar and you tried everything to treat your Hypo, it is much better to use this glucagon injection. Drinking orange juice, or eating a lump or cube of sugar sometimes does not do the trick to raise your blood sugar to at least within the range that you are expecting. When you tried everything to raise your blood sugar but to no avail, this glucagon injection is considered the emergency treatment for your hypo's, Low's or hypoglycemia. Always bear in mind that this glucagon injection needs prescription in order for you to keep it at home or carry it with you. It is also advisable for you to wear a medical alert tag or bracelet for anybody to identify yourself in case you will be found unconscious to be able to give you the right treatment you need. Glucagon shot can be given subcutaneously or intramuscularly.

Here are the following helpful tips on how you are going to use the glucagon injection either to yourself or to anyone who is diabetic. This is very important for you, your families, friends and relatives or loved ones to have the knowledge and practice in administering glucagon into your skin down to your muscles. In other words, Glucagon need to be administered intramuscularly to achieve the quickest and effective result. Glucagon solution is in pre filled syringe with needle. It comes in a kit and is ready to use. The accompanying instructions is very simple and easy to follow.

1. Read the label carefully, paying attention to the expiry date and the name of the glucagon itself making sure this is the right treatment you are going to receive.

2. Open the kit. Remove the needle cap.

3, Sometimes there is an air bubbles present inside the syringe. To remove this tiny bubbles you need to hold the syringe with its needle pointing in upright position. Push the plunger just enough to expel the air bubbles until it comes out of the very tip of the needle. Now you are ready to administer your Glucagon shot.

4. Look for the site where you need to inject the Glucagon. The muscles of the thighs and the upper arms are the most preferred site for this glucagon injection. If you are going to administer it to yourself, it is much easier to inject it to the thigh muscle. If you are going to administer this Glucagon shot to other person, you can either use the muscles of the thigh or the upper arm. Use the upper arm or the outer upper part of the thigh which shows a good amount of muscles. Do not inject it into your inner thigh because that is not the correct site.

5. using an alcohol swab wipe gently or clean the area to be injected. Hold or grasp gently the area by using your thumb and index finger and middle finger for an added support.

6. With your other hand, hold the glucagon syringe as if you are holding a pen to right on. In right angle position, administer the Glucagon shot into the skin down to the muscle.

7. Once the needle is in the muscle, withdraw the plunger for just a little, enough to see if there is a presence of back flow of blood into a syringe.

   The absence of back flow of blood indicates that you are in the right track. Now you are ready to push back the plunger and administer completely the glucagon solution into the muscles.

8. Once the glucagon had been administered completely, withdraw the syringe and needle from your skin and apply a gentle pressure to the injection site using an alcohol swab.

What about if you see a back flow of blood? What are you going to do about it? Simple. Just withdraw the needle completely and choose another site. The danger? You might hit a nerve that is really going to be painful if you continue pushing the glucagon injection. This is one reason why I don't personally recommend injecting intramuscular injection into your buttocks area because if you are not sure of what you are doing you might hit the sciatic nerve that may cause you to be paralyzed. Hitting the nerves is painful and at worst it could damage the nerves.

I want to share with you a real scenario that happened in a place where a patient was given an intra muscular injection in her buttock area in which a sciatic nerve was hit accidentally and the patient was not able to walk. To make story short, this patient was paralyzed. Although the injection given to this patient was not a glucagon shot, but just the same thing it is from intra muscular injection that damaged the sciatic nerve. So be careful.

Chapter X

ADHERING TO YOUR PRESCRIBED TREATMENT

Most of us are not fully aware of what is going on inside our body and what does our prescribed treatment really do inside our system. It seems that those prescribed medications are not really working. Have you ever wondered why those prescribed therapies won't help at all? In fact, your Physicians are really working hard and doing their best to help you treat your diabetes or most of all help your blood glucose level be kept under control. It is also possible that your Physicians are frustrated that your blood sugar could not be controlled no matter how hard they try to help you. Don't blame your Physician for the failure to control your diabetes. It is time to take your turn. You need to realize that you as a person has to be responsible to holistically follow the Doctor's prescriptions and advice in order to get the best result out of your prescribed medications. On top of this, you need to eat a healthy diet, avoid alcohol, stop smoking, get some exercise and keep monitoring closely your blood sugar maintaining it to as normal as possible. Without proper monitoring of your blood sugar, will put you at risk to a serious complications that will damage the different organs of your body.

Prescribed treatment must be adhered to so that a healthy quality of life must be maintained. A proper monitoring of blood sugar will help you decide to take action in case of any crisis that may occur. If your blood sugar is high, you need to take your prescribed insulin shots and/or take your diabetic pills on time. On the other hand, if your blood sugar is low, you must do the necessary action in order to fix it quickly.

Do not depend on insulin or pills as your treatment alone to fix your diabetes. Parts of the prescribed treatment your doctor will give you include exercise, quit smoking, avoidance of alcohol or take it in moderation and eating a healthy diet. Exercise will help you sweat out those toxins that are not needed in your body. It will also help you lose weight to prevent you from gaining unnecessary weight or obesity.

Do you smoke? Well. Smoking can be addicting too. To others, smoking is a habit, to some others it is just for a passing of time. Whatever the reasons are, smoking is not good to every body's health. It is a known fact that smoking is really bad to our overall health. It can even damage blood vessels and can cause high blood pressure. Did you ever tried to smoke and instead of inhaling it, blow it away onto your finger tip and you will see with your naked eyes the nicotine that you are getting from smoking your cigarette. It looks like a stain of brown rust and that is what you are getting that will damage your lungs and nerves, in which over a period of time, it will damage your overall health. If you could not quit smoking, talk to your Doctor who can help you for this.

There are people who has diabetes but they still continue to consume alcohol. Alcohol is not good for your health especially when taken in excess or consumed daily. Alcohol needs to be avoided or be only taken in moderation. According to American Diabetes association, drinking alcohol in an empty stomach can lower blood sugar.

Give love to yourself. Do not ignore your body needs. Give your body the best possible care it needs. Ignoring your body needs will put you into shock of critical illness that no one can be blamed except your very own self. Complete ignorance of our body needs will always be the leading role to a poor quality of life. I do believe that one of the leading causes of death worldwide is diabetes probably due to our complete ignorance of this kind of illness.

Adhering to the prescribed treatment is very important in managing your diabetes. Managing your diabetes is a very challenging job, yet it is just very easy if you are equipped with the knowledge and skill on how to do it. Keep reading this book and I can guarantee you that this will help you a lot in everyday life. The catch is: you will be proud of yourself in managing your diabetes in a most effective method and strategy. You will be surprised to discover that managing diabetes is easy as 1, 2, and 3. It is time to make a difference in your life.

Chapter XI

FOOT CARE

People who has diabetes are prone to have foot ulcer. There is also numbness due to poor blood supply to the extremities that they don't even feel their feet are already injured and when it is continuously unnoticed it becomes an ulcer in which this ulcer may become infected, not healing properly or will never heal at all.

Proper cleaning with mild soap and rinsing the feet with warm water as well as examining the whole feet regularly will reduce or prevent foot injury. A routine foot examination can be actually done every day while taking a bath or shower and after having a long walk. Never walk bare footed especially if you are diabetic because you are at high risk of foot injury.

Never cut corns or calluses by yourself to avoid injury, because when you injured yourself it will turn out to be an ulcer and can be a big and serious problem. The best thing to do is to see a professional health care providers who are well trained to remove calluses and corns. Your best choices are Diabetic nurse practitioners, Podiatrist, Chiropodist or even Registered nurses and Physicians. These are the qualified health care providers who can help you and assist you.

Exercise daily to improve the circulation of your feet. Exercise will not only improve foot circulation but it can also ease joint pain. Avoid crossing the legs while sitting because it can lead to decrease circulation, (Nursing procedure Made Incredibly Easy, 2002), or poor circulation to the lower extremities which includes the feet.

Always wear a well and properly fitted shoes to prevent pain, blisters, swelling and foot sores.

To sum it up, the following guidelines are recommended, (Nursing procedures, Made Incredibly easy, 2002):

1. Exercise daily

2. Wash feet with mild soap and warm water. Do not use hot water to avoid burning the skin.

3. Regular inspection of the skin of the feet for the presence of cuts, blisters, redness and swelling.

4. Shoes must fit properly.

5. Do not use harsh antiseptic to cuts, for example; iodine to prevent further tissue damage.

6. Always see a Doctor for advice to remove calluses or corns.

Most patients with diabetes has a very dry and flaky skin especially their lower extremities including the feet. A hypoallergenic and mild moisturizer is important for hydration of their skin. Moisturizer can be applied to the dry, flaky skin but it is not advisable to apply the moisturizer to the in between toes because these areas are usually moist. Dry skin is prone to cuts, blister formation and other skin injuries which of course, causes tissue damage; ulcer develops and becomes infected and gangrenous.

Cuts, blisters and other skin injuries will heal up very slowly or never heal at all when you have diabetes. It is always a smart choice to treat the skin injuries before infection sets in. It is clinically proven that an antibiotic treatment can prevent wound infection but it is unwise to use antibiotic all the time because it also causes your skin to be resistant to antibiotic. I recommend using a home remedy called Honey. It is proven that it can promote healing without the harmful effect of antibiotic.

When I was in the Middle East, I worked in a plastic surgery. Patient who are diabetic and undergone cosmetic surgery usually has a slow healing process of their surgery incision. There are also cases of slow wound healing process due to infection that sets in.

The plastic surgeon would apply honey to the wound bed and covered it with sterile dressing. It was done daily and you could see the difference on day 3 to day 5 that the wound improves. Amazingly, the healing is really quicker than expected and no signs of infection been observed in the wound. How powerful is this honey created by nature? Its healing power is so wonderful that few health care provider can notice its benefits in the world of medicine.

Another diabetic client has an infected foot ulcer. She was taking oral antibiotic at the same time an ointment antibiotic was applied to her foot wound. Due to her diabetes, the healing process of her wound was so slow. During her next visit to the Doctor's clinic she was scheduled to have debridement which means removing those necrotic tissues that were present on her wound. The necrotic tissues were not really bad so debridement was done as outpatient. After removing those dead tissues, the doctor poured honey into the wound bed and covered it with dressing. Every day, this Honey dressing was done in the doctor's clinic. Sometimes I do the dressing by myself. After a week, I noticed the a big difference in the appearance of the wound. It was actually a big improvement. The color of the wound bed and its surrounding areas appeared like a combination of bright red and pinkish. The purple and yellowish color of the dead tissues disappeared. It appeared that there was a good supply of blood to the cells which was evidence by the reddish and pinkish color of the wound bed. I was so excited and it was so interesting to know and observed those live tissues on that previously necrotic wound. I think the healing property of Honey contributed to the healing process of this once infected wound.

In UK England, I worked in one of the prestigious hospitals and my first job was in the Nursing Home. Most of my patients were diabetic. As expected, some of them has foot ulcer and bed sores. As I was taking my lunch break, I realized that the honey I was putting on my sandwich has a healing property. I even laughed silently at myself, thinking that I always put honey on my face especially when I have a skin breakdown and it was really very effective. Returning to my work area, I decided to put Honey on the foot ulcer of my patient and then I covered it with sterile dressing. I was doing this for straight two weeks every day. The fact that I was given the responsibility to take care of those patients who needs the correct wound dressing, I was able to take the opportunity to use Honey as a part of doing my wound care. At my own discretion, I found it easy to decide who needs honey dressing and to do this wound care procedure for the benefits of my patients who suffered from a long time foot ulcer that heals too slow. What a wonderful feeling that after a week or two the foot ulcer showed signs of big improvement. Again, this was due to the job well done not by myself alone, but by the Honey that I love to put in my sandwich. It is worth a try to use this Honey on your wound. But I will never advise you to eat Honey because it has an opposite impact on your diabetes and when you take it into your mouth it will increase your blood sugar. What I am talking here is that: Apply it directly into the wound bed but please do not put it into your mouth and eat it. Take it from me folks.

One day, I was surfing the internet when I came across a research about the health benefit of Honey. It was stated that a new study from one of the Universities in the United Kingdom of England that a Honey made solely from flowers found on the New Zealand manuka bush, inhibits several protiens, especially Fab I protein which is needed for biosynthesis. It is further stated, that MRSA infection may succumb to Honey due to its microbial effect of this New Zealand variety. As far as I can remember, this news release was on

September, 2009. Thanks to this amazing news. So the next time you need an antibiotic ointment for your wound, try this Honey. Cultured Honey can be used too. I used different kinds of Honey any way, and so far it still works for me. It is safer, affordable and your wound will heal quicker without any harmful side effects to your health.

In my present environment, I still see people with the same problem of foot ulcer. This means that wherever you are, foot injury could not be denied or ignored. The key here is prevention. Always pay close attention to your feet. Clean them every day, treat them with special care, and always give time and effort to examine your feet. Make your feet happy. Use a properly, well fitted foot wear. A happy feet make your whole being proud and happy too. Always remember that an ounce of prevention is better than a pound of cure. PREVENTION, PREVENTION, PREVENTION,

References and Reading

ALL-in-ONE., CARE PLANNING RESOURCE., MOSBY INC., 2004

American Diabetes Association, Inc., 1996

DR. Gomez, J., Living with diabetes

MERCK MANUAL OF MEDICAL INFORMATION, 2nd Home Edition, 2003

Nursing procedures, Made Incredibly Easy., Springhouse, PA., Springhouse Corp., 2002

Thibodeau and Patton., The Human Body in Health and Disease, 3rd ed., 2002.